Intermittent Fasting

Lose Weight, Get Fit and Add Years to Your Life With Intermittent Fasting

Sara Elliott Price

Published in The USA by:

Success Life Publishing

125 Thomas Burke Dr.

Hillsborough, NC 27278

Copyright © 2015 by Sara Elliott Price

ISBN-10: 1511850043

Disclaimer:

Every effort has been made to accurately represent this book and its potential. Results vary with every individual, and your results may or may not be different from those depicted. No promises, guarantees or warranties, whether stated or implied, have been made that you will produce any specific result from this book. Your efforts are individual and unique, and may vary from those shown. Your success depends on your efforts, background and motivation.

The material in this publication is provided for educational and informational purposes only and is not intended as medical advice. The information contained in this book should not be used to diagnose or treat any illness, metabolic disorder, disease or health problem. Always consult your physician or health care provider before beginning any nutrition or exercise program. Use of the programs, advice, and information contained in this book is at the sole choice and risk of the reader.

Table of Contents

Chapter 1:

Introduction to Intermittent Fasting

Intermittent Fasting is increasing in popularity and is becoming the preferred dieting method as more and more people discover it. It is practiced by people wanting to burn fat, gain muscle, and improve their health in general. In this book we will discuss in detail what Intermittent Fasting is, how it works, the benefits it offers, its psychological and hormonal effects, different types of Intermittent fasts, as well as answer some frequently asked questions about it. By the time you finish reading this book, you will have a clear idea about what Intermittent Fasting is, and how to get started right away.

Fasting

Fasting is a religious and spiritual practice that has been practiced by people for hundreds of years. Every year, during the month of Ramadan, Muslims all over the word fast for an entire month by not eating or drinking anything from sunrise to sunset. The reasons for fasting are many, from pleasing a God to giving your stomach a rest. Research has shown that there are many benefits to Intermittent Fasting and that it, indeed, does help you lose weight and gain muscle. The results of Intermittent Fasting vary from person to person.

1

What is Intermittent Fasting?

The term 'intermittent' is used for things occurring at irregular intervals of time. When combined with fasting, Intermittent Fasting, it is used to describe a dietary plan in which the people practicing it alternate between fasting and not fasting. According to research, it has been found that people who consume less calories are healthier and live longer than those who eat more. Intermittent Fasting is based on the same idea. The goal is to incorporate a fast or fasts weekly, to lose excess weight, increase certain hormones, such as HGH and to increase the detoxification of the body.

Now, when you think about Intermittent Fasting and not eating for a day, it might sound impossible to you. That is very natural, and, in fact, people believe that fasting intermittently will make them weak. However, that is not true at all. If that were the case, Intermittent Fasting would have become obsolete by now, like several other dieting methods in the past. In the age of science, anything that makes big claims is researched, studied, and investigated by scientists, and they lay the truth bare in front of everyone. So, if Intermittent Fasting were not actually beneficial, we would have known it by now. But the research that has been put out has already proven otherwise.

A lot of research has been put into food consumption and it has been proven that people who limit their intake of food also have a decreased risk of getting diseases. Diets usually prove to be very difficult because you have to constantly limit your calorie intake and avoid almost all of your favorite, delicious, calorie-rich foods. We are all human beings and we usually slip or cheat, and even if we don't diet plans are simply too hard and demanding to stick to. Intermittent Fasting, however, easily takes care of that problem.

Now most diet plans ask you to stick to a certain diet no matter what, but we know that we are all human beings and we are not all the same. A one-size-fits-all approach is not going to work for everyone, it can't. But there are different types of Intermittent Fasts, and there is going to be one that you will enjoy. If you do not know which one to go for, you can simply try out all the methods available until you find the one that suits you.

Intermittent Fasting is becoming a preferred method because people are okay with feeling very hungry for a period of time (Intermittent Fast), instead of feeling hungry all the time, as is the case with diet plans. A sharp pang of pain that lasts for a small period of time is better than a continuous but low pain.

It is a crude example, yes, but it should give you an idea about how Intermittent Fasting may feel, and the only difference is that instead of pain, you will feel a little hungry for a few hours. When you fast, a process called 'autophagy' takes place in your body. It removes the damaged and dead cells from your body and makes sure your tissues and blood stay clean.

Now there are different types of Intermittent Fasts, from daily to weekly, and we will discuss all of them in full detail in later chapters. So, whichever style of fasting intermittently you choose, your time will be divided into two basic periods: (a) Fasting, and (b) Not Fasting (Eating). During the Not-Fasting (Eating) period, you will be free to eat whatever you want, as much as you want. During the Fasting period, you will abstain from eating food.

IF Is Natural
Intermittent Fasting is very natural, and it might be surprising for you to know that all of us already practice it. When we sleep, which is usually 8 hours, we are fasting as well. We are doing it naturally, and we benefit from it.

The benefits it gives us when we are sleeping can also be achieved when we are awake. It has been practiced in the past, has worked well, and is still in practice today. In fact, our ancestors would go through times of feast and famine. They would be forced to fast intermittently, which means living this lifestyle is in your genes.

Now that you have a basic idea of what Intermittent Fasting is, we will move on to how and why it works in the following chapters. It is important to understand how it works and what benefits you are going to experience. We will also include a guide on how to start Intermittent Fasting.

Chapter 2:

Intermittent Fasting Works

As mentioned before, several studies have shown that if people reduce their calorie intake by up to forty percent, their life span will increase. The studies conducted on animals like rodents and fruit flies show that if their calorie intake is reduced, their life span is increased by about 33% or more. Many studies have been conducted on Intermittent Fasting and its results, most of them have ruled in favor of IF. Researchers tend to agree that limiting your food and calorie intake does prevent a lot of diseases in people as they grow older and promotes a healthy life in general.

The recent research that has focused on Intermittent Fasting, an alternate way of controlling the calorie intake, found it promising. There is evidence in favor of this type of fasting that supports the fact that Intermittent Fasting provides the same benefits as other dieting methods of controlling calorie intake, if not more.

Intermittent Fasting is done in different was from not eating for certain periods of time daily to multi-day fasts. As said before, it is preferred because instead of controlling the calorie intake 24/7, people practicing this method of calorie intake only need to control it for a selected few hours. In addition to that, research conducted on rodents found that the rodents who ate one day and skipped eating the next day consumed fewer calories than they would if they ate on both days. Another study found that Intermittent Fasting reduces the risk of getting diabetes.

When we fast, our cells defend us more actively against molecular damage. Fasting intermittently makes our body more responsive to insulin, a hormone that regulates the blood sugar levels in our body, which is a very good thing, because when this responsiveness is decreased, the risk of diabetes, heart failure, and obesity is increased. The animals and human beings who live long lives have been found to have low levels of insulin in their bodies because the cells in their body are more sensitive to insulin.

Research studies conducted on mice that are kept on an intermittent fasting diet have found that feeding these mice exclusively fatty foods during the not-fasting/eating periods does not increase obesity rates. Yet, mice on a regular eating schedule fed the same number of calories and same type of food experience a large increase in obesity rates. This goes on to show how Intermittent Fasting prevents obesity.

There are two things that happen to us daily that make us eat. The first thing is that we eat when we are hungry, and that is okay. The second thing is that we eat when we 'think' we are hungry, and that is not good. There are times when we are really hungry and we eat a lot of food, more than we needed to, because it takes time for the body to send the signal to the brain that it is full. And, usually, before the signal is sent, we have already consumed more food than required. For this, it is suggested that people should eat slowly. Eating slowly makes sure that you do not end up overeating. But, in today's fast paced word, no one has time to slow down their eating.

We have started living our lives systematically, sleeping at a fixed time, going to work and following a schedule in everything, except eating. But if we make eating a part of our schedule too, then we can prevent ourselves from overeating, like the Intermittent Fasting method that gives you an eight-hour window daily for eating. You can eat however much you want, whenever you want during these eight hours, after which your fasting period begins. When this period ends, you are actually hungry, and since you have avoided calories for 16 hours, it is okay for you to eat whatever you want.

Some weight loss experts argue that eating whatever you want does not help with weight loss. So, in that case, they suggest Intermittent Fasting, but add that while you do not have to fully control the calorie intake, it will help increase your weight loss if you do not indulge in overeating. Some people practicing Intermittent Fasting claim to have lost over 20 pounds in just a few months with no other changes to diet or exercise. How well Intermittent Fasting works depends entirely on the individual and how much they eat during the not-fasting/eating period.

Some people have a faster metabolism than others, so two people can fast intermittently in the same way, eat the same things, and still end up with different results. But one thing is for sure, that whether you lose fat fast or slowly, you do lose fat when fasting intermittently, so even if you do not see the results immediately, there is nothing to worry about, because you will see the results eventually, albeit it might take you a bit longer. You can also add exercise to your routine to boost the weight loss and improve your health, and if your workout happens to be in your fasting period, just make sure that you are well hydrated and you will be good to go. Water, after all, is your go to beverage during Intermittent Fasts.

Chapter 3:

Why Intermittent Fasting

Whatever method of dieting you choose, they all work the same way. The goal is to give your body less calories than it needs, so that your body turns to its fat reserves when it needs energy. When your body needs energy, it will first burn your excess sugar and after the sugar is gone it will turn to the fat stores in your body, and the result will be weight loss.

The more fat you burn, the healthier you become. Once you have reached your ideal weight, you just have to make sure that you do not consume calories in excess of what your body needs.

To be more precise about Intermittent Fasting, we can say that it is not a diet. In fact, it is a dieting schedule, which increases your fat loss and improves protein synthesis and hormone production in your body, thus keeping and growing lean muscle becomes easier. Normally when the body needs energy, it turns to the food that we have eaten. With intermittent fasting you allow your body to burn through all your sugar so it has no choice but to burn body fat for energy.

According to Mark P. Mattson, an expert on fasting and someone who has observed and studied intermittent fasting in both human beings and animals, we are physiologically able to handle intermittent fasting because it dates back to the eating patterns of our ancestors', back when food was not available all the time or in abundance. According to him, we are genetically programmed to go hungry for longer stretches than we currently do. This goes to show that intermittent fasting is not just a modern technique but something that is already wired or programmed into our body, so naturally we are better able to handle intermittent fasts as compared to other methods of dieting for weight loss.

It has also been observed that when people fast intermittently, they slowly start eating less during their not-fasting/eating periods. Even though they are already fasting for a period of time, when allowed to eat, they get less hungry. This further aids in weight loss and improving health.

Now, as mentioned earlier in this chapter, one of the reasons we overeat is because we think we are hungry, when in fact, we are not. When fasting intermittently, people learn to differentiate between the two. Because when they observe fasting periods, they understand clearly whether they are actually hungry or not. Sometimes people think they are hungry because they have developed a habit of eating at a certain time, and at other times, it is just thirst mistaken for hunger.

According to a study that was published in the International Journal of Obesity, it was found that the women who were over-weight and consumed 650 calories a day, two times a week, and about 2500 calories on other days, were able to lose fourteen pounds in just six months. When compared to women who consumed 1500 calories per day, it was found that the latter only lost 12 pounds in the same amount of time. The women who lost more weight were actually eating 3300 more calories per week than the women who ate less. This just goes to show how fasting for even short amounts of time increase the amount of fat the body burns.

Intermittent Fasting may be difficult in the beginning because it takes some time to get used to it. The body can take anywhere from 5 days to 2 weeks to get adjusted to it, but once it does, it is totally worth it.

The Intermittent Fasting approach is very heavily promoted to the athletic community so that they can easily achieve and maintain a lean and strong body. When compared to the benefits of other controlled calorie intake diets, Intermittent

Fasting leads to decreased fat mass, allays discomfort caused by low energy, improves the cellular sensitivity to insulin, as well as improves the blood lipid profiles.

The key to the success of a weight loss plan lies in how well it can be maintained. People can stick to diet plans for some time but then they give up. In comparison, it is found that it is easier for people to follow the Intermittent Fasting approach. Since it is also genetically programmed into us, not only is it easier for us but is also something that we can actually maintain.

When considering a long-term diet, Intermittent Fasting is definitely something that needs to be considered. When starting a weight loss plan, you have to ask yourself if this is something that you can do for life. Constantly controlling your calorie intake will also mean that you will miss out on a lot of things, but Intermittent Fasting ensures that you get the best of both worlds.

How IF Burns Fat

When you look at it from the fat burning point of view, you will notice how powerful an approach it is. When your body is well fed, it produces insulin so that your blood sugar is maintained at a safe level. The job of insulin is to transfer the extra glucose from the blood to the muscles, fat cells, and liver for storage, and while doing so, it increases fat storage as well. This is controlled when fasting intermittently.

How IF Improves Metabolism

Some people argue that fasting intermittently slows down your metabolism and is not good for you. That is not true, because if we look back to our ancestors', again, we will notice that back in those days, they never had food all the time, which means they were not able to feed themselves all the time. As a result of which, it is natural for the body to go hungry, or on fasts, and it does not harm your metabolism at all. In fact, it is good for it.

Chapter 4:

Benefits of Intermittent Fasting

The benefits of Intermittent Fasting are too many to count, and only those who practice it regularly really know exactly how they've personally benefited, but, in this chapter, we will cover the main benefits of Intermittent Fasting.

We keep hearing about how healthy it is to have six small meals every day, but that also means we get extra calories on a regular basis and that our body continuously stores fat. It is not really known where the idea of having six small meals came from, but there is no scientific evidence that supports it. However, Intermittent Fasting is scientifically supported.

Another logic behind Intermittent Fasting is that when we follow this approach, our body does not have to spend a lot of resources and time on functions that consume too much energy, like digestion. So, when it is not spending time on digestion, it saves energy that it can then spend on performing other functions in our bodies that benefit us in other ways. Consuming 6 meals daily prevents that from happening by keeping the body busy on digestion almost all the time. When all these things are considered together, Intermittent Fasting puts our body in a state that is ideal for losing weight and also prevents diseases.

Detoxification

Our body is constantly cleaning and detoxifying itself. We do not have to eat something special or go on a special diet for detoxification. The many cellular processes that take place in our body also take a toll on the cells in our body, resulting in damaged and dead cells, which are automatically cleansed in a process called autophagy. Now, even though this process is happening all the time all by itself, what we eat also plays a role.

If our diet is very poor, this process is significantly hindered and detoxification slows down. And when we are eating all the time, the body spends most of its energy and resources on digesting that food and slows down the detoxification process. But when we are fasting intermittently, we are giving our body ample time to detoxify. It also slows down the aging process of the body and prevents Alzheimer's Disease.

Weight Loss

When we consume calorie rich foods, our body does not immediately use up all the sugar or glucose it needs from the food. Instead, it stores it in the liver in the form of glycogen. The liver only has a limited capacity for storing glycogen, and when its capacity is filled, the rest of it is stored in the form of fat. When the body needs energy, the first place it turns to will be the liver.

The body uses up its supply of glycogen from the liver in about 8 hours, and after that it will turn to the fat stores for energy. But if you eat six meals a day, before the 8 hours are up and before your body can turn to the cells and start burning fat for energy, it gets more food than it can use, so it leaves the fat stores as is. But when you fast intermittently, say, for 16 hours, your body gets time to use up all the glycogen and then turns to fat stored in the body. This is how Intermittent Fasting aids in weight loss.

Hormone Regulation

Intermittent fasting has many effects on hormones. It dramatically impacts the levels of growth hormones in humans. The increased levels of Human Growth Hormone improve endurance and also speed up the repairing of muscles, while slowing down the aging process at the same time. According to a recent study, interval training when fasting intermittently found that Human Growth Hormone in men was increased by 2000% and in women by 1300%.

Insulin Levels

Intermittent Fasting normalizes insulin activity. We have already discussed the effects of insulin earlier so we will not go into further detail here.

Mental Effects

Intermittent Fasting also has mental benefits. It leaves people feeling light and active. Creative people like artists and writers often fast so that they can continue working without disturbing their workflow. Intermittent Fasting gives you a sense of inner peace, stability, energy, and strength.

Reduced Hunger

When you start practicing Intermittent Fasting, it may be hard in the beginning and you may find yourself eating more during your non-fasting/eating periods. However, once you get used to it, you will start eating less during your non-fasting periods. As a result, your calorie consumption will decrease automatically.

Better Focus

When you're fasting, your body produces beneficial hormones that improve your concentration and focus. Your quality of work and life in general are improved because you have a clear mind.

More Energy

When you start fasting intermittently, as opposed to eating all the time, your body becomes stable internally. As a result of this, your body has more energy all the time.

How to Get the Most from Intermittent Fasting

To make the most of Intermittent Fasting, the trick is to not try too hard. Select your intermittent fasting routine, stick to your schedule, and enjoy what you eat. You should try to eat healthy foods, not only while fasting intermittently but also in general. While you do not necessarily need to count calories all the time, you should avoid junk food. The point of intermittent fasting is to go with the flow, take it easy, and not to push yourself too hard so that you can actually maintain this lifestyle for a long time.

Chapter 5:

How to Get Started Fast

As I said earlier, we live our lives very systematically. Intermittent Fasting is a system for eating, a schedule, that we can incorporate into our daily lives and reap the benefits. To make it simple, Intermittent Fasting is a dieting pattern where you choose not to eat for a certain period of time, regularly; the period can be daily or weekly, whatever suits you.

For instance, a person fasting daily would choose to eat during an 8-hour window, and will abstain from eating for the remaining 16 hours of the day. It might sound difficult, but if you sleep for 8 hours, then you basically only have to abstain from eating for 8 hours. It is very easy, healthy, and practical.

To start fasting intermittently, all you need to do is decide how you want to fast, when you want to fast, and then get started. The Intermittent Fasts are mainly divided into two types. They are:

- **Long Intermittent Fasts**
- **Short Intermittent Fasts**

Long Intermittent Fasts

During the long intermittent fasts, you do not fast too often, perhaps once in a week or two, as you see fit, but the fasts are longer, for up to 24 hours.

Short Intermittent Fasts

The short intermittent fasts are of smaller durations and are kept more often, like every day or every other day.

It is entirely up to you to decide which method of fasting you want to go with. It is best if you try both, because one may sound easier to you, but trying both will tell you for sure which one is actually easy for you and which one you actually want to go with.

In the next chapter we will discuss the different types or styles of Intermittent Fasting.

Chapter 6:

Different Types of Fasting

There are various different types of Intermittent Fasts, from the standard ones to custom ones. I will explain them all in this chapter. They include:

- Eat Stop Eat / Long Intermittent Fasts (24 hours)
- Leangains Method / Daily Fasts (14 - 16 hours)
- The Warrior Diet / Partial Daily Fast (20 hours)
- Fat Loss Forever / Hybrid Fast (A mixture of all three)
- Alternate-Day Fasting

Eat Stop Eat (Long Intermittent Fast) (24 Hours)
Eat Stop Eat is the intermittent fasting method for healthy eaters and was started by Brad Pilon.

How To:
Using this method, you fast for exactly 24 hours once or twice in a week or two. In simple words, you take a 24-hour break from eating, or, as Brad Pilon calls it, 24 break from eating. During this time, you do not eat anything at all, but you are free to consume calorie free beverages if you want. And when

the 24 hours are up, you can return to eating like you normally do. So, for instance, if your last meal was at 8PM on Saturday and you begin your fast, then you will not be eating anything until 8PM on Sunday, at which time your fast will end and you can go back to eating normally.

It is best that when your fasting period ends, instead of having a huge meal, you stick to regular sized meals, as if you weren't fasting at all. Adding a workout to your fasting routine ensures that you will make the most of it. You can take some time to get used to Eat Stop Eat, so you can start by fasting for shorter intervals and slowly increase them until you are able to fast for 24 hours. Moreover, if they are very difficult for you, you can allocate an hour in which you eat during the fast, say after 12 hours are completed. Secondly, you can incorporate these fasts in your routine however you want. So, if you adjust them in such a way that the last 8 hours are the same as your sleeping hours, you will basically only fast consciously for 16 hours and yet reap the benefits of a full 24-hour fast.

Leangains Method (Daily Fasts 14 - 16 Hours)
This method of fasting is for people go to the gym regularly and are trying to build muscle and lose fat and was started by Martin Berkhan.

How To:

The fasting period for men and women is different when using the Leangains method. For men, the fasting period is 16 hours, and for women the fasting period is 14 hours.

According to this method, you have an 8-10 hour window for eating, depending on your gender, and you abstain from eating during the remaining 14-16 hours. During your fasting period, you avoid all foods that have calories.

It is ideal to begin this fast at night so that the time you spend sleeping is also taken in to account, though you cannot have breakfast immediately after waking up, unless your 14, or 16, hours are up. After fasting this way for a few days, you will get a general idea of how it is working for you, and then you can change your timing to make the most of it and to make it convenient for yourself.

It is important to maintain a proper eating window when fasting using this method to ensure that you eat as much as you need. If you incorporate a workout in your fasting routine, then you have to watch what you eat too. On days you work out, you'll need to eat more carbohydrates. It is recommended that you eat three times during your 8-10 hour eating window.

The Warrior Diet (Partial Daily Fast) (20 Hours)

This method of Intermittent Fasting is for the people who are devoted and like following rules and was started by Ori Hofmekler.

How To:

If you want to be a warrior and follow the Warrior Diet plan, then you will be expected to fast for 20 hours daily and have a big, nutritious meal at night. The reasoning behind this method of fasting is that human being are actually nocturnal eaters, so by consuming a large meal at night daily, you feed nutrients to the body in sync with the circadian rhythms of the night.

Since the fasting period is very long, the warriors are not supposed to abstain from food completely. They can have fresh juices, uncooked vegetables, protein servings, etc. if they want. According to Ori Hofmekler, this method maximizes the Sympathetic Nervous System's 'fight or flight' response. It boosts energy, promotes alertness, and burns fat. During the four-hour eating window, warriors can overeat to maximize the Parasympathetic Nervous System's ability to help the body heal and become relaxed and calm. It also allows the body to repair itself and promotes growth during this time. The best thing about this method is that you can have a few snacks during your fasting period, which makes it very easy for you to fast. The production of hormones also increases in the body during the day.

Fat Loss Forever (Hybrid Fast)

This method of fasting combines different parts of all three methods mentioned above. It is designed for people that go to the gym regularly and enjoy cheat days as well. It was started by John Romaniello and Dan Go.

How To:

This plan can be purchased from fatlossforever.net. This is a fasting plan that incorporates elements from all other fasting plans and also includes a cheat day, which is followed by a 36-hour fasting period. Further details of this plan can be found on the website. This type of fasting is said to increase your productivity and improve your focus and concentration, along with weight loss.

Alternate-Day Fasting

This method of fasting is for disciplined dieters who have a certain weight goal they want to achieve. James Johnson, M.D, started this method.

How To:

In this method of fasting, you eat normally one day and eat only a little the next, and so on. The days when you eat less are called your low-calorie days, and on these days you can only consume 1/5th of the calories you normally consume. So, if you are a woman and your normal calorie intake is 2000 calories, on your low-calorie day, you will only consume 400 calories; if you are a man and your normal calorie intake is 2500 calories, on your low-calorie day, you will only consume 500 calories. When you start fasting using this method, you can initially use meal replacements, but after 2 weeks, you have to start eating normal foods only, even during your low-calorie days.

Now, if you want, you can follow any one of these methods, or experiment with them till you find the one that suits you the best. All of them promote weight loss, though some are faster than the others, but your goal is to stick to a method that you can stick to for a long time.

Chapter 7:

Food Recommendations

Although there are no restrictions on the foods that you can eat when fasting intermittently, you should incorporate healthy food like fruits, and vegetables into your diet. Following are some foods that promote weight loss and health:

Avocado:

Avocados contain vitamins C, E, and B6, omega 9 fatty acids, and iron, potassium, magnesium, and niacin. They have high fiber content, and although they are high in fat, they have oleic acid in them which suppresses hunger. You should have a quarter or half an avocado daily to start burning your fat.

Banana

A banana contains 92 calories on average. It has a great taste and is rich in fiber. It makes a delicious and energy packed snack. When buying bananas, buy the ones that have a shade of green on the peels. You can have a banana daily for a quick energy boost.

Chili

Chili contains a chemical called capsaicin. Capsaicin starts the fat burners in the body and boosts weight loss. Chili can also suppress your cravings for sweet and calorie rich foods, so it should be incorporated in your diet when you want to lose weight.

Fig

A piece of fig only contains 45 calories and 0.2 grams of fat. Figs are also packed with energy and can help with weight loss because of their low calorie content. They make great stomach fillers, and can be eaten along with other fruits as well.

Papaya

A serving of papaya only contains 20 calories. When it is dried, it retains its sweet taste. There is an enzyme found in papaya that aids the body in breaking down the proteins; the enzyme is called papain. A papaya contains 1% of the daily-recommended calorie intake, so it is suggested that you incorporate papayas into your diet when trying to reduce your calorie intake.

Tomato

One ounce of sun-dried tomatoes has only 70 calories in them, and one gram of fat. Although they have high sugar content and should be avoided by people who have diabetes, others seeking to lower their calorie intake can eat them. They are rich in potassium, vitamin A, copper, and manganese. Moderately eating sun-dried tomatoes does not lead to any weight gain.

Almonds

Almonds help regulate the blood sugar levels. One of the reasons for weight gain is abnormal blood sugar levels, but eating almonds can prevent this. Almonds have antioxidant properties and are rich in nutrients. They also have the unique ability to block calories. It was found that almonds have a composition of cell walls that can block calories so that they do not get absorbed by the body. Replace crackers with almonds in your low calorie meals.

Pistachio (Skinny Nuts)

Pistachios are called skinny nuts because of their low calorie content. You can eat 30 pistachios and only gain 100 calories. A study found that people who incorporated pistachios in their diet were able to lose 12 pounds of weight in just three months. They contain soluble fiber and phytosterols, and both of them help lower the levels of bad cholesterol in the body.

Green Tea

Green Tea is the world's most famous drink, because it has numerous benefits and aids in weight loss. It is good for your skin, strengthens your immune system, and it has a great taste. Research has found that the people who exercise and drink green tea as well are able to lose twice as much weight as those who exercise but do not drink green tea. It has anti-oxidant properties as well. To maximize the effects of green tea, it should be taken at least three times a day. It is a great drink to have after meals, and in the morning before breakfast. It has a refreshing taste and is available in a wide variety. To further give it a boost for losing weight, squeeze half a lemon into it. Honey can also be added to sweeten it.

Vegetable Juices

Vegetable juices are gaining popularity nowadays and a lot of people prefer a vegetable cocktail instead of water. We already know vegetables are low in fat content and are almost always very low in calories. When talking about vegetable juices, the best ones are the ones that are leafy and green. You do not have to stick to a particular vegetable juice recipe.

Just pick up a few of your favorite vegetables, put them in a blender, and prepare yourselves a vegetable smoothie. You can experiment with them until you find a combination that you love. They are power packed and good for your hair and skin too. They are also a great way to detox and cleanse your body.

Turmeric

Turmeric is a spice common in India. It not only aids in weight loss but also helps in maintaining it afterwards. It can be added to the meals you make to ensure that your body does not start storing fat. Like almonds, turmeric is also able to block fat. You can use turmeric or turmeric powder in your meals for flavor. According to researchers, one and a half tablespoons of turmeric every day is ideal for people trying to lose weight. It also lowers cholesterol and can keep depression away. In Japan, turmeric is used for treating hangovers. You can get your daily dose of turmeric from supplements as well.

Chapter 8:

Frequently Asked Questions

Who is Intermittent Fasting for?

Intermittent Fasting is for anyone wanting to gain muscle and lose fat, and become healthy in general.

Which methods of Intermittent Fasting should I use?

There are several different methods of Intermittent Fasting. The method you should go for is the one that you find to be the easiest. Since you need to stick to a fasting plan for hopefully a lifetime, you need to make sure it's convenient and doable for you. You can try and experiment with different methods until you find the one that you want to stick to.

When does my period of fasting start?

This is one of the most common questions people ask. Suppose you start eating your lunch at 2pm and finish at 3pm, your fasting period will start as 3pm. Simply put, your fast starts the moment you stop eating food.

What about breakfast?

If your fasting schedule is such that your breakfast time coincides with your fast, you can still have breakfast if you want. It is okay to have anything that is less than 50 calories, so you can add a bit of milk to your tea or cream to your coffee. Just make sure that you do not exceed the 50 calories. As long as you consume less than 50 calories, your body will remain in a state of fast.

When should I eat during my not-fasting window?

I suggested that you should have three meals during your 8 hour not-fasting/eating window, but that is not a hard and fast rule. You can eat whenever you want during that period. Three meals are suggested to ensure that you get enough food so that you can easily make it through the next 14, or 16, hours.

Can I exercise while fasting?

Yes, you can exercise while you are fasting. Just make sure that you are well hydrated. During the days when you plan to work out, try to get some carbs to increase your energy, so that you can work out properly. Workouts, especially for weight loss, have great results when you are fasting intermittently, because the body is already in a state of burning fat, and when you add exercise to this, the fat burn is practically doubled.

What if I can't fast for that long?

No matter which Intermittent Fasting method you go with, it's going to be difficult in the beginning. To get used to it, you can fast for shorter intervals, and have a snack while fasting. Just remember that small fasts and snacks are only to make it easy for you to begin fasting. In a week or two, you should be able to fast properly without snacks.

When will I see results?

Since Intermittent Fasting is not a diet but a controlled way of eating, it can take up to 6 months for you to get significant results. But since the goal is to continue fasting for a long time, for over 6 months, you will be pleased with the results.

Anything else I should know?

The only thing you need to remember when fasting is to take it easy. You're going to be fasting for a long time, so you need to make it a habit. Take your time to get used it, relax, and don't force yourself. If one method is too difficult, try another. If you can't fast for long, perhaps try alternate-day fasting.

Thanks for reading! If you're looking for a great diet that goes perfectly with intermittent fasting be sure to check out my book 'Paleo Diet for Beginners: Lose Weight, Feel Great & Start Thriving Living the Paleo Lifestyle.'